OVERCOMING SCLERODERMA

How to Manage Symptoms, Psychology Effects, Diagnosis, Finding Solutions and Reversing Scleroderma

Dr.Rebecca J. Reynolds

CONTENT

INTRODUCTION

The Journey to Overcoming Scleroderma

Chapter 1

What Is Scleroderma

    Forms of scleroderma

    Understanding the Causes

Chapter 2

Signs and Symptoms of Scleroderma

    Skin Involvement

    Internal Organ Involvement

    Raynaud's Phenomenon

    Gastrointestinal Symptoms

    Respiratory Issues

    Joint and Muscle Pain

Chapter 3

Diagnosis and Medical Evaluation

    The Diagnostic Process

Chapter 4

Managing Scleroderma Symptoms

    How is scleroderma managed

    Treating scleroderma.

        Exercise.

shared defense.

Diet.

Tooth care.

handling of stress.

sleeping and resting properly.

consuming a balanced diet.

finding ways to manage your fears and anxieties.

Chapter 5

Exercise plan for people living with Scleroderma

30 Days Exercise Plan For You

MEAL PLAN

Conclusion:

Navigating Scleroderma with Courage and Hope

INTRODUCTION

Welcome to "OVERCOMING SCLERODERMA: How to Manage Symptoms, Psychological Effects, Diagnosis, Finding Solutions, and Reversing Scleroderma." This book is a beacon of knowledge, support, and inspiration for individuals and their loved ones facing the challenges of scleroderma.

Scleroderma is a complex and rare autoimmune disorder that affects the skin, blood vessels, and internal organs. It can bring physical discomfort, emotional upheaval, and significant lifestyle adjustments. However, this book is here to tell you that there is hope, and you are not alone on this journey.

In these pages, we will embark on a comprehensive exploration of scleroderma, from understanding its nature and diagnosis to finding ways to manage its symptoms and cope with its psychological effects. We will delve into treatment options and potential breakthroughs on the horizon. Most importantly, we will discuss the concept of reversing scleroderma, a topic that holds promise for many individuals facing this condition.

Each chapter of this book is designed to equip you with knowledge, tools, and strategies to not only cope with scleroderma but to thrive in spite of it. We will address the physical, emotional, and practical aspects of living with this autoimmune disease, providing you with insights into how to regain control over your life.

You'll discover inspiring stories of individuals who have successfully navigated the challenges of scleroderma, proving that it is possible to overcome even the most daunting obstacles. Throughout this journey, remember that you are a scleroderma warrior, resilient and capable of facing whatever lies ahead.

Whether you are someone newly diagnosed, a longtime scleroderma fighter, or a family member seeking to understand and support a loved one, this book is your guide, your ally, and your source of hope. Together, we will explore the path toward better management, improved well-being, and the potential for reversing scleroderma.

Let us embark on this journey of overcoming scleroderma, armed with knowledge, determination, and the unwavering belief that a brighter future is within reach.

The Journey to Overcoming Scleroderma

The journey to overcoming scleroderma is not a solitary path but a collective effort, encompassing the strength of individuals, the support of loved ones, and the guidance of healthcare professionals. It's a journey marked by challenges, resilience, and a relentless pursuit of a better quality of life. In this chapter, we'll explore what this journey entails and the key elements that play a crucial role in navigating it successfully.

Understanding the Complexity: Scleroderma is a complex autoimmune disease that affects each individual differently. It involves the immune system mistakenly attacking healthy tissues, leading to the hardening and tightening of the skin, blood vessel damage, and potential involvement of internal organs. Understanding the nature of this condition is the first step in the journey.

Diagnosis and Uncertainty: Many individuals with scleroderma face a period of uncertainty before receiving a definitive diagnosis. We'll discuss the diagnostic process, the role of healthcare providers, and the importance of early detection.

Managing Symptoms: Scleroderma presents a wide range of symptoms, from skin changes to gastrointestinal issues and joint pain. Effective management of these symptoms is essential for improving daily life and overall well-being.

Psychological Effects: The emotional impact of scleroderma should not be underestimated. Anxiety, depression, and stress often accompany the physical symptoms. We'll explore the psychological effects of the disease and strategies for coping with them.

Treatment Options: While there is no cure for scleroderma, various treatment options are available to manage symptoms and slow disease progression. We'll discuss medications, physical therapy, and lifestyle modifications.

Hope for Reversal: One of the most exciting aspects of the scleroderma journey is the emerging research and potential for disease reversal. We'll delve into the latest developments in this area and share stories of individuals who have experienced remission.

Support Systems: A robust support system is invaluable when facing scleroderma. We'll explore the role of family, friends, and support groups in providing emotional and practical support.

Advocacy and Awareness: Advocating for yourself and raising awareness about scleroderma can make a significant impact. We'll discuss ways to advocate for better care and share information about scleroderma with the broader community.

As we embark on this journey together, remember that you are not alone. Countless individuals have faced scleroderma with courage and determination, and their experiences can inspire and guide you. The journey to overcoming scleroderma may be challenging, but with knowledge, support, and hope, it is a journey you can navigate successfully.

Chapter 1

What Is Scleroderma

Scleroderma is an uncommon but chronic autoimmune condition in which dense, thick fibrous tissue replaces healthy tissue. The immune system typically aids in the body's defence against illness and infection. Scleroderma patients' immune systems cause other cells to overproduce the protein collagen. This excess collagen is deposited in the organs and skin, causing thickening and hardness (a process akin to scarring).

Scleroderma can affect the gastrointestinal tract, lungs, kidneys, heart, blood vessels, muscles, joints, and skin, though it typically just affects the skin. In its most extreme forms, scleroderma can be fatal.

Forms of scleroderma

There are 2 major forms of scleroderma, localized and systemic. Systemic scleroderma can be broken down into two main types: diffuse and limited.

Localized scleroderma

The more common form of the disease, localized scleroderma, affects only a person's skin, usually in just a few places. It often appears in the form of waxy patches or streaks on the skin, and it is not uncommon for this less severe form to go away or stop progressing without treatment.

Diffuse scleroderma

As its name implies, this form affects many parts of the body. Not only can it affect the skin, but it also can affect many internal organs, hindering digestive and respiratory functions, and causing kidney failure. Systemic scleroderma can sometimes become serious and life-threatening.

Limited scleroderma

Also known as CREST syndrome, each letter stands for a feature of the disease:

C alcinosis (abnormal calcium deposits in the skin).
R aynaud's phenomenon (see the symptoms section).
E sophageal dysmotility (difficulty swallowing).
S clerodactyly (skin tightening on the fingers).
T elangectasias (red spots on the skin).
Patients with limited scleroderma do not experience kidney problems. The skin thickening is restricted to the fingers, hands and forearms, and also sometimes the feet and legs. Digestive involvement is confined mostly to the esophagus. Among later complications, pulmonary hypertension, which can develop in 20% to 30% of cases, can be potentially serious. In pulmonary hypertension, the arteries from the heart to the lungs narrow down and

generate high pressure on the right side of the heart, which can ultimately lead to right sided heart failure. Early symptoms of pulmonary hypertension include shortness of breath, chest pain, and fatigue.

Understanding the Causes

Scleroderma is a complex autoimmune disease with an intricate web of causes that researchers are still unraveling. While the exact cause remains elusive, several factors are believed to contribute to the development of this condition. In this section, we'll explore these factors and delve into the current understanding of what may trigger scleroderma.

Autoimmune Origins: Scleroderma is classified as an autoimmune disease, which means that the immune system, which normally protects the body from harmful invaders, mistakenly attacks its own healthy tissues. In the case of scleroderma, this immune dysfunction leads to inflammation and fibrosis (the thickening and scarring of tissues).

Genetic Predisposition: Genetics is thought to play a role in the development of scleroderma. While the disease is not directly inherited, there appears to be a genetic predisposition. Research suggests that certain genes may make some individuals more susceptible to scleroderma when exposed to specific environmental triggers.

Environmental Triggers: Environmental factors are believed to be key triggers for scleroderma in genetically predisposed individuals. These triggers can vary and may include exposure to toxins, infections, or other external factors. However, identifying specific triggers can be challenging due to the complex and multifactorial nature of the disease.

Immune System Dysfunction: Scleroderma involves a dysregulated immune system, where immune cells and antibodies mistakenly target healthy tissues, particularly the connective tissues. This immune response leads to the hallmark symptoms of skin tightening and damage to internal organs.

Vascular Abnormalities: Vascular abnormalities are commonly observed in individuals with scleroderma. Damage to blood vessels can contribute to the disease process, affecting circulation and leading to symptoms such as Raynaud's phenomenon, where the fingers and toes turn white or blue in response to cold or stress.

Role of Fibrosis: In scleroderma, the excessive production of collagen—a protein that provides structural support to tissues—results in fibrosis. This fibrosis causes tissues to become stiff and lose their elasticity, leading to the characteristic skin changes and potential internal organ involvement.

It's important to note that while these factors are associated with the development of scleroderma, the interplay between them remains a subject of ongoing research. Scleroderma is a complex and heterogeneous disease, meaning it can manifest differently in each individual. Understanding its causes is just one piece of the puzzle on the journey to overcoming this condition.

Chapter 2

Signs and Symptoms of Scleroderma

Skin Involvement

One of the most distinctive and visible features of scleroderma is its impact on the skin. Skin involvement is often an early sign of this autoimmune disease and can vary widely in severity and presentation among individuals. In this chapter, we'll explore the signs and symptoms of scleroderma related to skin, understanding the changes that may occur and how they can affect daily life.

1. Skin Tightening: Scleroderma's hallmark symptom is the tightening and hardening of the skin. This tightening can occur gradually and typically affects the fingers, hands, face, and forearms. As the skin loses its flexibility, it can restrict movement and lead to a sensation of stiffness.

2. Thickened and Shiny Skin: Affected skin may become thicker, shinier, and less pliable than normal. This can give the skin a waxy or stretched appearance.

3. Skin Discoloration: Scleroderma can cause changes in skin color, ranging from pale or white patches (hypopigmentation) to reddish or purplish areas (telangiectasia) due to the dilation of tiny blood vessels near the skin's surface.

4. Ulcerations: In severe cases, the tightness and reduced blood flow to the fingers and toes can lead to digital ulcers. These are painful sores or open wounds that may be prone to infection.

5. Facial Changes: Scleroderma can affect the face, leading to tightness around the mouth and limited mouth opening. This can impact speech, eating, and facial expressions.

6. Raynaud's Phenomenon: Many individuals with scleroderma experience Raynaud's phenomenon, which causes the fingers and toes to turn white, blue, or purple in response to cold temperatures or stress. When blood flow returns, they may become red and tingly.

7. Nail Abnormalities: Changes in the nails are common in scleroderma and may include nail fold (periungual) telangiectasia, cuticle thickening, and distortion of nail shape.

It's important to note that scleroderma's skin involvement can vary from person to person. Some individuals may experience only mild symptoms, while others may have more extensive skin changes. Additionally, skin involvement is often just one aspect of the disease, as scleroderma can also affect internal organs, leading to a wide range of symptoms.

Internal Organ Involvement

Scleroderma is a multifaceted autoimmune disease that can extend beyond skin-related symptoms to affect various internal organs and systems within the body. In this section, we'll delve into the signs and symptoms of internal organ involvement in scleroderma, highlighting the importance of early detection and management.

Gastrointestinal Symptoms:

Esophageal Dysfunction: Many individuals with scleroderma experience difficulty swallowing (dysphagia) due to reduced esophageal motility. This can lead to heartburn, regurgitation, and an increased risk of aspiration pneumonia.

Gastrointestinal Motility Disorders: Scleroderma can disrupt the normal movement of the gastrointestinal tract, causing symptoms such as bloating, diarrhea, constipation, and abdominal pain.

Interstitial Lung Disease:
Scleroderma-associated interstitial lung disease (ILD) involves scarring and inflammation of lung tissue. It can result in breathlessness, a persistent cough, and decreased lung function.

Pulmonary Hypertension: Pulmonary hypertension (PH) is high blood pressure in the arteries of the lungs. In scleroderma, PH can strain the right side of the heart and cause symptoms like shortness of breath and fatigue.

Scleroderma Renal Crisis: Although rare, scleroderma renal crisis is a severe complication characterized by a sudden increase in blood pressure and kidney dysfunction. Symptoms may include headaches, confusion, and decreased urine output.

Cardiac Manifestations:

Pericarditis: Inflammation of the pericardium (the sac surrounding the heart) can lead to chest pain and discomfort.

Arrhythmias: Irregular heart rhythms, such as atrial fibrillation, can occur in scleroderma and may cause palpitations and dizziness.

Musculoskeletal Involvement:

Joint Pain: Scleroderma can cause joint pain and inflammation, often in the hands and fingers. This can affect mobility and daily activities.

Other Organ Systems:

Eye Involvement: Dry eyes, inflammation, and other eye problems can occur in some individuals with scleroderma.

Endocrine Abnormalities: Hormonal imbalances and thyroid dysfunction are possible in scleroderma.

It's crucial to recognize that not all individuals with scleroderma will experience internal organ involvement, and the severity can vary widely. Regular medical monitoring and communication with healthcare providers are essential for early detection and intervention.

Managing internal organ complications in scleroderma may involve medications to reduce inflammation, improve lung function, or control blood pressure. In some cases, individuals may require specialized treatments or interventions, such as lung transplantation or medications for pulmonary hypertension.

Raynaud's Phenomenon

Raynaud's phenomenon is a hallmark sign of scleroderma and one of the most recognizable symptoms associated with this condition. It is characterized by episodic color changes in the fingers, toes, or sometimes other extremities, such as the nose or ears. In this section, we will explore Raynaud's phenomenon, its connection to scleroderma, and its impact on those living with this autoimmune disease.

Understanding Raynaud's Phenomenon: Raynaud's phenomenon is a vascular disorder that affects the small blood vessels in the extremities. It typically occurs in response to cold temperatures or emotional stress, leading to a sequence of color changes in the affected digits:

White Phase: During an episode of Raynaud's, the fingers or toes turn white as blood flow to the area is significantly reduced. This phase, known as the vasoconstrictive phase, can cause numbness and a sensation of cold.

Blue Phase: After the white phase, the affected digits may turn blue or purple due to insufficient oxygen supply. This phase is a result of prolonged vasoconstriction.

Red Phase: As the episode subsides or when the fingers or toes are warmed, blood flow gradually returns, causing the digits to turn red. This phase is marked by a tingling or throbbing sensation.

Raynaud's in Scleroderma:
Raynaud's phenomenon is particularly prevalent in individuals with scleroderma. In fact, it is often one of the earliest signs of the disease. In scleroderma-related Raynaud's, the condition tends to be more severe and longer-lasting compared to primary Raynaud's phenomenon, which occurs on its own without an underlying autoimmune condition.

Impact on Daily Life:
Raynaud's can significantly impact the quality of life for individuals with scleroderma. The episodes of color changes and associated discomfort can make it challenging to perform

everyday tasks, especially in cold environments. Simple activities like holding a cold drink or typing on a keyboard can trigger Raynaud's episodes.

Management and Coping:
Managing Raynaud's phenomenon in scleroderma involves a combination of lifestyle changes and medication. Lifestyle modifications may include keeping extremities warm, wearing gloves or mittens in cold weather, and avoiding cold exposure whenever possible. Medications, such as vasodilators, may be prescribed to help improve blood flow and reduce the frequency and severity of episodes.

Understanding Raynaud's as a sign and symptom of scleroderma is essential for early diagnosis and management.

Gastrointestinal Symptoms

Gastrointestinal (GI) symptoms are common in individuals with scleroderma and can significantly impact daily life. In this section, we'll explore the GI symptoms associated with scleroderma and how they manifest as signs of the disease.

1. Gastroesophageal Reflux Disease (GERD): GERD is a prevalent GI symptom in scleroderma. It occurs when stomach acid flows back into the esophagus, causing heartburn, chest pain, and regurgitation. The tightening of the lower esophageal sphincter due to scleroderma-related fibrosis contributes to GERD.

2. Dysphagia: Scleroderma can lead to difficulty swallowing, a condition known as dysphagia. Individuals may experience a sensation of food getting stuck in the throat or chest. Dysphagia can result from esophageal muscle dysfunction and tissue scarring.

3. Gastroparesis: Gastroparesis is a condition where the stomach muscles do not function properly, causing delayed emptying of the stomach. This can lead to symptoms such as bloating, early satiety (feeling full quickly), and nausea. Gastroparesis in scleroderma is often attributed to nerve damage affecting the GI tract.

4. Small Intestinal Bacterial Overgrowth (SIBO): SIBO occurs when there is an excessive growth of bacteria in the small intestine. This can lead to symptoms like abdominal pain, diarrhea, and malabsorption of nutrients. Scleroderma-related intestinal changes can contribute to SIBO development.

5. Bowel Dysfunction: Scleroderma can affect the lower GI tract, leading to symptoms such as chronic constipation, diarrhea, or alternating episodes of both. These bowel issues can result from abnormalities in gut motility.

6. Fecal Incontinence: Some individuals with scleroderma may experience loss of bowel control, known as fecal incontinence. This can be distressing and may occur due to weakened sphincter muscles.

7. Nutritional Challenges: Due to the various GI symptoms, individuals with scleroderma may face nutritional challenges, including difficulty in maintaining a well-balanced diet and absorbing essential nutrients. This can lead to weight loss and nutritional deficiencies.

It's crucial for individuals with scleroderma to communicate these GI symptoms with their healthcare providers promptly.

Respiratory Issues

Respiratory issues are among the wide range of signs and symptoms that individuals with scleroderma may experience. Scleroderma can affect the respiratory system in various ways, leading to both mild and severe respiratory complications. In this section, we will explore the respiratory symptoms associated with scleroderma and their impact on individuals living with this condition.

1. Shortness of Breath: Shortness of breath, also known as dyspnea, is a common respiratory symptom in scleroderma. It may occur due to several factors, including lung fibrosis (scarring of lung tissue) and inflammation of the lung lining (pleuritis). As lung function declines, individuals may find it increasingly difficult to breathe during physical activity and, in severe cases, even at rest.

2. Cough: Persistent coughing is another respiratory symptom frequently observed in scleroderma. This cough can be dry or produce phlegm and may be linked to lung inflammation or irritation caused by fibrosis.

3. Reduced Lung Capacity: Scleroderma can lead to a reduction in lung capacity. The scarring of lung tissue can limit the expansion and contraction of the lungs, resulting in decreased lung function. This reduced capacity may lead to a feeling of breathlessness.

4. Interstitial Lung Disease: Interstitial lung disease (ILD) is a term used to describe various lung conditions characterized by inflammation and scarring of the lung tissue. ILD is a common complication of scleroderma and can result in symptoms such as cough, shortness of breath, and reduced oxygen levels in the blood.

5. Pulmonary Hypertension: Scleroderma-associated pulmonary hypertension (PH) is a serious complication that affects the blood vessels in the lungs. It can lead to increased pressure in the pulmonary arteries, causing symptoms such as shortness of breath, chest pain, and fatigue.

6. Aspiration: Scleroderma can affect the muscles involved in swallowing, leading to an increased risk of aspiration—when food, liquid, or saliva enters the airways instead of the stomach. Aspiration can result in lung infections and respiratory symptoms.

7. Raynaud's Phenomenon: While primarily a vascular symptom, Raynaud's phenomenon, common in scleroderma, can also affect the respiratory system. Raynaud's can cause blood vessels in the lungs to constrict, potentially leading to decreased blood flow and oxygen supply to the lungs.

It's important to note that respiratory issues can vary widely among individuals with scleroderma. Some may experience mild symptoms, while others may face more severe complications.

Joint and Muscle Pain

Among the common manifestations of scleroderma are joint and muscle pain, which can significantly impact an individual's quality of life. In this section, we'll explore these symptoms and their implications in the context of scleroderma.

Joint Pain (Arthralgia):
Joint pain, often referred to as arthralgia, is a common symptom experienced by many individuals with scleroderma. It can affect various joints throughout the body, including the fingers, wrists, knees, and shoulders. Joint pain in scleroderma is typically characterized by:

Achy Discomfort: Individuals often describe the pain as a persistent, dull ache in the affected joints.
Morning Stiffness: Joint stiffness, particularly in the morning or after periods of inactivity, is a frequent complaint.

Reduced Range of Motion:
Scleroderma-related joint pain can limit joint mobility and make it challenging to perform daily activities.
The exact cause of joint pain in scleroderma is not fully understood, but it is believed to result from inflammation and immune system dysfunction. It's important to differentiate between scleroderma-related joint pain and other forms of arthritis, as the treatment approaches may vary.

Muscle Pain (Myalgia):
Muscle pain, known as myalgia, is another symptom that individuals with scleroderma may experience. This pain typically affects the muscles of the arms, legs, and torso. Myalgia in scleroderma may present as:

Muscle Tenderness: The affected muscles can become tender to the touch, and pressing on them may elicit discomfort.
Weakness: Some individuals may also experience muscle weakness, which can impact their ability to perform physical tasks.

Chronic Discomfort: Muscle pain in scleroderma can be chronic, with episodes of exacerbation and remission.

Chapter 3

Diagnosis and Medical Evaluation

The Diagnostic Process

Scleroderma can be difficult to diagnose. Scleroderma may initially be mistaken for lupus or rheumatoid arthritis because it can affect other areas of the body, such as the joints.

Your doctor will conduct a thorough physical examination following a discussion of the medical history of your immediate family. He or she will be on the lookout for any of the aforementioned symptoms, particularly any thickening or hardening of the skin around the fingers and toes or any skin discoloration. If scleroderma is suspected, tests will be ordered to confirm the diagnosis, as well as to determine the severity of the disease. These examinations could consist of:

Blood tests: 95% of scleroderma patients have elevated levels of immune factors called antinuclear antibodies.
Testing for these antibodies in prospective scleroderma patients can help with an accurate diagnosis even though they are also present in other autoimmune diseases like lupus.

Tests of pulmonary function are performed to gauge how well the lungs are working. Verifying whether or not scleroderma has spread to the lungs, where it can result in the formation of scar tissue, is critical if the condition is suspected or has already been diagnosed.
Lung damage may be evaluated using an X-ray or computed tomography (CT scan).

Electrocardiogram: Scleroderma can result in scarring of the heart's tissue, which can cause congestive heart failure and irregular heartbeats.
To determine whether the disease has affected the heart, this test is carried out.

To check for complications like pulmonary hypertension and/or congestive heart failure, an echocardiogram (a heart ultrasound) is advised once every 6 to 12 months.

Gastrointestinal tests: In addition to the intestine's walls and muscles, scleroderma can also affect the esophagus.
In addition to causing heartburn and making it difficult to swallow, this can hinder the absorption of nutrients and the transit of food through the intestines.
A procedure known as an endoscopy, which involves inserting a small tube with a camera on the end, is occasionally used to view the esophagus and the intestines.
Manometry is a test that assesses the strength of the esophageal muscles.

Kidney function: When scleroderma affects the kidneys, the effects can include an increase in blood pressure and the leakage of protein into the urine.
A sudden rise in blood pressure may occur in its most severe form (known as scleroderma renal crisis), which can lead to kidney failure. Blood tests are one way to evaluate kidney function.

Chapter 4

Managing Scleroderma Symptoms

How is scleroderma managed

Scleroderma does not have a current treatment. Instead, the focus of treatment is managing and controlling the symptoms.

In order to effectively treat and manage scleroderma, which can have a wide range of symptoms, a combination of methods is frequently required.

Skin treatments: Topical drugs are frequently helpful for localized scleroderma.
Both to treat hardened skin and to stop the skin from drying out, moisturizers are used.
Nitrates, such as nitroglycerin, are prescribed to increase blood flow so that finger sores can heal.
Because nitrates relax the smooth muscles, the arteries dilate (widen).
The smooth muscles are what support some internal organs and blood vessels in most cases.
It's important to discuss with your doctor whether or not nitrates may be appropriate for you because they can cause side effects like nausea, dizziness, rapid heartbeat, and blurred vision.

Digestive remedies: A range of medications may be prescribed to assist patients with heartburn and other digestive issues.
Proton pump inhibitors (such as Prevacid, Protonix, or Nexium) and H 2 receptor blockers (such as Zantac or Pepcid) are a few examples of over-the-counter and prescription antacids that fall into this category.
The mechanism by which proton pump inhibitors function is to stop the stomach's acid pump from releasing stomach acid. H 2 receptor blockers function by inhibiting histamine, a body chemical that encourages the production of stomach acid.

Treatment of lung disease: A recent NIH study has shown that the chemotherapy drug cyclophosphamide (Cytoxan®) is effective in treating patients with scleroderma who have pulmonary fibrosis (scarring of the lung tissue) that is rapidly worsening.
In patients with interstitial lung disease who also had scleroderma, this study demonstrated how well oral cyclophosphamide could improve lung function and quality of life.

The most effective treatment for pulmonary hypertension is a continuous pump-assisted intravenous infusion of the prostaglandin epoprostenol (Flolan®).

Treprostinil (Remodulin®), a related prostaglandin, can be infused subcutaneously as an alternative.

Prostaglandins are hormone-like substances produced by the body that, among other things, aid in smooth muscle relaxation and, as a result, blood vessel dilation.

FDA-approved treatments for pulmonary hypertension include oral bosentan (Tracleer®), sildenafil (Revatio®), and inhaled iloprost (Ventavis®).

Both severe (drug-refractory) interstitial lung disease and pulmonary hypertension may be treated with lung transplantation.

Joint issues: Anti-inflammatory medications may be prescribed for scleroderma patients who experience joint issues.

Inflammation, which causes pain and swelling, is reduced by these medications. Physical therapy can occasionally be beneficial in preventing joint contraction.

Vasodilators like calcium channel blockers (Procardia® or Norvasc®), nitroglycerin patches/ointment, alpha blockers, and sildenafil are effective treatments for Raynaud's phenomenon.
Aspirin and other antiplatelet medications are frequently added.
Oral medications like sildenafil (Viagra®) or bosentan (Tracleer®) used as a preventative measure can be helpful for ischemic digital ulcers.
A trial of intravenous epoprostenol (Flolan®) or alprostadil should be conducted while the patient is hospitalized for fingers with severe ulceration or impending gangrene.
Local wound care and a long course of the proper antibiotics are required for infected ulcers.

There is no known cure for Sjögren's syndrome, but the symptoms can be managed.

Artificial tears and cyclosporine eye drops
(Restasis®) can be used to treat dry eyes.
Drinking liquids or chewing gum can help with
dry mouth.
The use of saliva-stimulating medications, such
as Evoxac® or Salagen®, may be advised for
more severe cases of dry mouth.

Scleroderma-related kidney issues can be
managed and treated with medication,
particularly Angiotensin Converting Enzyme
(ACE) inhibitors, as well as dialysis, depending
on the severity of the condition.

Treating scleroderma.

There are many actions a person with
scleroderma can take to better manage the
condition, in addition to taking prescribed
medications correctly and consistently.
Among them are:.

Exercise.

Regular exercise will not only help you feel better physically and spiritually, but it will also help keep your joints flexible and increase circulation.
For recommendations on suitable exercises, speak with your physician or physical therapist.

shared defense.

Avoid heavy lifting and labor-intensive tasks when your joints are in pain to prevent further damage.
You can learn new techniques from a physical therapist to carry out regular tasks without putting too much stress on your joints.

skin defense.

The symptoms of Raynaud's phenomenon as well as the dry, thick patches of skin that are caused by localized scleroderma can both benefit from taking the proper precautions and caring for your skin. There are numerous ways to do this, including:.

Make sure to dress appropriately during the colder months.
Boots, a hat, gloves, and a scarf will keep your body warm and shielded from the cold, and these items will also aid in maintaining circulation and keeping the blood vessels in your extremities open.

Put on numerous, thin layers.
Rather than wearing one heavy layer, these will keep you warmer.

To keep the blood flowing to your feet, put on comfortable shoes or boots.

Install a humidifier in your home to help maintain the humidity level.

Utilize soaps and creams that are especially formulated for dry skin.

Diet.

In addition to eating nutritious foods to get the right amounts of vitamins and nutrients, it's critical to eat foods that won't make pre-existing stomach issues worse.
There are several ways to do this, including:.

foods that cause heartburn should be avoided.

drinking water or another liquid to further soften food.

consuming foods high in fiber to reduce constipation.

eating more frequent, smaller meals as opposed to three large ones.
As a result, the body is able to digest the food more quickly.
Wait at least four hours before lying down after a substantial meal.

Place some bricks or blocks underneath your bed to raise the head by about six inches. This will stop stomach acid from penetrating the esophagus while you're sleeping.

Tooth care.

Getting the right dental care is crucial for people with scleroderma and Sjögren's syndrome.
Cavities and tooth decay are more likely to develop when Sjögren's syndrome is present.

handling of stress.

It's critical to learn how to manage or reduce stress because it has the potential to affect many different aspects of your health and wellbeing, including your blood flow.
The actions listed below can be used to achieve this:.

sleeping and resting properly.

Avoiding stressful situations when possible.

consuming a balanced diet.

finding ways to manage your fears and anxieties.

Exercising.

Scleroderma does not yet have a known cause or treatment, but it is frequently a manageable, slowly progressing condition that allows its sufferers to live healthy, active lives.
The best methods for managing scleroderma and lowering the risk of new complications, as with many other conditions, are community support groups and education about the condition.

Chapter 5

Exercise plan for people living with Scleroderma

Exercising with scleroderma requires careful planning and adaptation to individual needs and limitations. Consult with your healthcare provider before starting any exercise program to ensure it's safe and suitable for your specific condition. Here's a general exercise plan for people living with scleroderma:

Warm-Up:

Begin with a gentle warm-up to prepare your body for exercise. This can include slow walking, marching in place, or gentle arm circles.
Duration: 5-10 minutes.
Stretching:

Perform gentle stretching exercises to improve flexibility. Focus on major muscle groups. Hold each stretch for 15-30 seconds, and repeat 2-3 times for each muscle group. Stretching can help alleviate stiffness associated with scleroderma.

Strength Training:

Include low-intensity strength training exercises to maintain muscle strength and joint stability. Use resistance bands, light weights, or your body weight for resistance.
Perform 1-2 sets of 10-15 repetitions for each exercise.
Focus on exercises for the arms, legs, and core.

Cardiovascular Exercise:

Engage in low-impact aerobic activities to improve cardiovascular health and endurance. Options include walking, stationary biking, swimming, or water aerobics.

Start with 10-15 minutes and gradually increase the duration as tolerated.
Aim for 30 minutes of cardiovascular exercise most days of the week.

Balance and Coordination:

Balance exercises can help prevent falls and improve coordination.
Practice standing on one leg, heel-to-toe walking, or using stability balls.
Include these exercises 2-3 times per week.

Breathing Exercises:

Scleroderma can affect lung function, so include breathing exercises to maintain lung capacity.
Practice deep breathing, pursed-lip breathing, and diaphragmatic breathing.
Incorporate these exercises into your routine daily.

Cool-Down:

Finish your exercise session with a gentle cool-down to gradually lower your heart rate and reduce muscle tension.
Gentle stretching or relaxation exercises can be part of your cool-down.
Duration: 5-10 minutes.

Listen to Your Body:

Pay close attention to your body's signals. If you experience pain, fatigue, or discomfort, stop or modify the exercise.
Stay hydrated throughout your workout.
Rest when needed and avoid pushing yourself too hard.

Adaptations:

Adapt exercises based on your individual limitations and symptoms.
Modify the intensity, duration, and type of exercise as needed.

Consider working with a physical therapist who can create a tailored exercise program.

Consistency:

Consistency is key to reaping the benefits of exercise. Aim for regular, manageable workouts.

Keep a journal to track your progress and make adjustments as necessary.
Remember that the goal of exercise with scleroderma is to improve overall fitness, maintain joint mobility, and enhance your quality of life. Prioritize safety, consult your healthcare provider, and be patient with yourself as you progress on your exercise journey.

30 Days Exercise Plan For You

Week 1: Gentle Movements

Day 1:

Warm-up: Begin with five minutes of slow, deep breathing exercises.
Exercise: Gentle neck stretches (side-to-side, forward and backward).
Cool-down: Finish with five minutes of relaxation and deep breathing.

Day 2:

Warm-up: Five minutes of slow, deep breathing.
Exercise: Seated leg lifts, 2 sets of 10 repetitions per leg.
Cool-down: Five minutes of relaxation and deep breathing.

Day 3:

Warm-up: Five minutes of deep breathing.
Exercise: Seated marching in place, 2 sets of 10 repetitions per leg.
Cool-down: Five minutes of relaxation and deep breathing.

Day 4:

Warm-up: Five minutes of deep breathing.
Exercise: Seated seated arm curls using light weights or resistance bands, 2 sets of 10 repetitions.
Cool-down: Five minutes of relaxation and deep breathing.
Day 5:

Warm-up: Five minutes of deep breathing.
Exercise: Seated torso twists, 2 sets of 10 repetitions per side.
Cool-down: Five minutes of relaxation and deep breathing.
Day 6 and Day 7: Rest or Gentle Walking

Week 2: Flexibility and Balance

Day 8:

Warm-up: Five minutes of deep breathing.
Exercise: Seated ankle circles, 2 sets of 10
repetitions per leg.
Cool-down: Five minutes of relaxation and deep
breathing.
Day 9:

Warm-up: Five minutes of deep breathing.
Exercise: Seated heel-to-toe stretches for
balance, 2 sets of 10 repetitions per leg.
Cool-down: Five minutes of relaxation and deep
breathing.
Day 10:

Warm-up: Five minutes of deep breathing.
Exercise: Seated hip stretches, 2 sets of 10
repetitions per leg.
Cool-down: Five minutes of relaxation and deep
breathing.
Day 11:

Warm-up: Five minutes of deep breathing.

Exercise: Seated side leg lifts for hip strength, 2 sets of 10 repetitions per leg.
Cool-down: Five minutes of relaxation and deep breathing.
Day 12:

Warm-up: Five minutes of deep breathing.
Exercise: Seated seated leg extensions, 2 sets of 10 repetitions per leg.
Cool-down: Five minutes of relaxation and deep breathing.
Day 13 and Day 14: Rest or Gentle Walking

Week 3: Strengthening

Day 15:

Warm-up: Five minutes of deep breathing.
Exercise: Standing supported wall push-ups, 2 sets of 10 repetitions.
Cool-down: Five minutes of relaxation and deep breathing.
Day 16:

Warm-up: Five minutes of deep breathing.

Exercise: Standing seated squats (use a chair for support), 2 sets of 10 repetitions.
Cool-down: Five minutes of relaxation and deep breathing.
Day 17:

Warm-up: Five minutes of deep breathing.
Exercise: Standing calf raises, 2 sets of 10 repetitions.
Cool-down: Five minutes of relaxation and deep breathing.
Day 18:

Warm-up: Five minutes of deep breathing.
Exercise: Standing bicep curls using light weights or resistance bands, 2 sets of 10 repetitions.
Cool-down: Five minutes of relaxation and deep breathing.

Day 19:

Warm-up: Five minutes of deep breathing.
Exercise: Standing leg raises for hip strength, 2 sets of 10 repetitions per leg.

Cool-down: Five minutes of relaxation and deep breathing.
Day 20 and Day 21: Rest or Gentle Walking

Week 4: Putting It All Together

Day 22:

Warm-up: Five minutes of deep breathing.
Exercise: Perform a combination of seated stretches, standing balance exercises, and gentle strength training exercises for a total of 20-30 minutes.
Cool-down: Finish with five minutes of relaxation and deep breathing.
Day 23-28:

Continue the routine from Day 22, gradually increasing the duration of your exercises as tolerated.

Day 29 and Day 30: Rest or Gentle Walking

Remember that the key to this exercise plan is to progress gradually and listen to your body. If you experience pain, discomfort, or worsening symptoms, consult your healthcare provider.

MEAL PLAN

Creating a nutritious and balanced meal plan for individuals living with scleroderma is essential to support overall well-being and manage symptoms. Here's a meal plan with a variety of recipes, including instructions, ingredients, dessert ideas, smoothies, and more:

Day 1 - Breakfast:

Meal: Scrambled eggs with spinach and tomatoes.
Ingredients: Eggs, fresh spinach, diced tomatoes.

How to Make: Whisk eggs, sauté spinach and tomatoes, add eggs, cook until set.

Day 1 - Lunch:

Meal: Grilled chicken breast with quinoa and steamed broccoli.

Ingredients: Chicken breast, quinoa, broccoli.

How to Make: Grill chicken, cook quinoa, steam broccoli.

Day 1 - Dinner:

Meal: Baked salmon with a side of asparagus and brown rice.

Ingredients: Salmon fillet, asparagus, brown rice.

How to Make: Bake salmon, roast asparagus, cook brown rice.

Day 2 - Breakfast:

Meal: Greek yogurt parfait with honey and mixed berries.

Ingredients: Greek yogurt, honey, mixed berries.

How to Make: Layer yogurt, berries, and honey.

Day 2 - Lunch:

Meal: Lentil soup with a side salad.

Ingredients: Lentils, vegetables, mixed greens.

How to Make: Prepare lentil soup, toss mixed greens for the salad.

Day 2 - Dinner:

Meal: Grilled shrimp with quinoa and sautéed spinach.

Ingredients: Shrimp, quinoa, spinach.

How to Make: Grill shrimp, cook quinoa, sauté spinach.

Day 3 - Breakfast:

Meal: Oatmeal with sliced banana and chopped nuts.

Ingredients: Oats, banana, nuts (almonds or walnuts).

How to Make: Cook oats, top with banana and nuts.

Day 3 - Lunch:

Meal: Chickpea salad with mixed greens and balsamic vinaigrette.

Ingredients: Chickpeas, mixed greens, balsamic vinaigrette.

How to Make: Combine chickpeas, mixed greens, and drizzle with vinaigrette.

Day 3 - Dinner:

Meal: Baked cod with steamed broccoli and quinoa.

Ingredients: Cod fillet, broccoli, quinoa.

How to Make: Bake cod, steam broccoli, cook quinoa.

Day 4 - Breakfast:

Meal: Whole-grain waffles with Greek yogurt and fresh berries.

Ingredients: Whole-grain waffles, Greek yogurt, fresh berries.
How to Make: Toast waffles, top with yogurt and berries.
Day 4 - Lunch:

Meal: Mixed bean and vegetable chili with whole-grain crackers.
Ingredients: Mixed beans, vegetables, whole-grain crackers.
How to Make: Prepare chili, serve with crackers.
Day 4 - Dinner:

Meal: Grilled tofu with roasted Brussels sprouts and sweet potato.
Ingredients: Tofu, Brussels sprouts, sweet potato.
How to Make: Grill tofu, roast vegetables.
Day 5 - Breakfast:

Meal: Smoothie with spinach, banana, unsweetened almond milk, and protein powder.

Ingredients: Spinach, banana, almond milk, protein powder.

How to Make: Blend ingredients until smooth.

Day 5 - Lunch:

Meal: Caprese salad with fresh tomatoes, mozzarella, basil, and balsamic glaze.

Ingredients: Tomatoes, mozzarella, basil, balsamic glaze.

How to Make: Layer ingredients and drizzle with balsamic glaze.

Day 5 - Dinner:

Meal: Baked chicken breast with sautéed green beans and brown rice.

Ingredients: Chicken breast, green beans, brown rice.

How to Make: Bake chicken, sauté beans, cook brown rice.

Day 6 - Breakfast:

Meal: Whole-grain toast with avocado spread and poached eggs.

Ingredients: Whole-grain bread, avocado, eggs.

How to Make: Toast bread, spread avocado, top with poached eggs.

Day 6 - Lunch:

Meal: Spinach and quinoa salad with roasted beets and goat cheese.

Ingredients: Spinach, quinoa, roasted beets, goat cheese.

How to Make: Toss ingredients and serve.

Day 6 - Dinner:

Meal: Grilled salmon with sautéed kale and quinoa.

Ingredients: Salmon fillet, kale, quinoa.

How to Make: Grill salmon, sauté kale, cook quinoa.

Day 7 - Breakfast:

Meal: Overnight oats with chia seeds, almond milk, sliced banana, and a drizzle of honey.

Ingredients: Oats, chia seeds, almond milk, banana, honey.

How to Make: Combine ingredients and refrigerate overnight.

Day 7 - Lunch:

Meal: Caprese salad with fresh tomatoes, mozzarella, basil, and balsamic glaze.

Ingredients: Tomatoes, mozzarella, basil, balsamic glaze.

How to Make: Layer ingredients and drizzle with balsamic glaze.

Day 7 - Dinner:

Meal: Baked chicken breast with sautéed green beans and quinoa.

Ingredients: Chicken breast, green beans, quinoa.

How to Make: Bake chicken, sauté beans, cook quinoa.

This meal plan provides a variety of nutrient-rich options to support individuals living with scleroderma.

Conclusion:

Navigating Scleroderma with Courage and Hope

In the intricate tapestry of human health, scleroderma stands as a complex and enigmatic challenge. This autoimmune disease, with its diverse symptoms and uncertain causes, tests the strength and resilience of individuals and their loved ones. Yet, within the labyrinth of scleroderma's complexities, there is courage, hope, and the unwavering spirit of those who refuse to be defined by their diagnosis.

In our exploration of scleroderma, we have journeyed through its many facets, from understanding its causes and the diagnostic process to managing its symptoms and grappling with its psychological effects. We've delved into the treatments and therapies that offer relief, and we've glimpsed the promise of research that may one day lead to the reversal of this condition.

Throughout this journey, the individuals living with scleroderma have emerged as true warriors. They've faced uncertainty with determination, pain with resilience, and challenges with unwavering hope. Their stories have illuminated the path forward, proving that life with scleroderma can be vibrant, meaningful, and fulfilling.

While scleroderma may be part of an individual's story, it does not define their entire narrative. The journey of living with scleroderma is marked by victories, both large and small, and the constant pursuit of a better quality of life. It is a journey of adaptation, where individuals learn to adjust to new realities while holding fast to their dreams and aspirations.

As we conclude our exploration of scleroderma, let us carry with us the knowledge that the human spirit is unbreakable. Scleroderma may present formidable challenges, but it also reveals the extraordinary strength within each person who faces it. It reminds us of the power of resilience, the importance of hope, and the value of a supportive community.

To those living with scleroderma, you are not alone on this journey. You are surrounded by a network of healthcare professionals, loved ones, and fellow warriors who stand beside you. Together, we look forward to a future where the mysteries of scleroderma are unraveled, where treatments continue to advance, and where the hope of reversal becomes a reality.

As we close this chapter, may the courage and hope that define the scleroderma community inspire us all to face life's challenges with unwavering determination.

Together, we move forward, embracing each day with strength, resilience, and the belief that a brighter, healthier future is within reach.